Gisele Senhorini

Speech Therapy and Aphasia

Gisele Senhorini

Speech Therapy and Aphasia

Analysis of a subject's therapeutic process

ScienciaScripts

Imprint

Cover image: www.ingimage.com

This book is a translation from the original published under ISBN 978-3-330-76824-6.

Publisher:
Sciencia Scripts
is a trademark of
Dodo Books Indian Ocean Ltd. and OmniScriptum S.R.L publishing group

120 High Road, East Finchley, London, N2 9ED, United Kingdom
Str. Armeneasca 28/1, office 1, Chisinau MD-2012, Republic of Moldova, Europe
Managing Directors: Ieva Konstantinova, Victoria Ursu
info@omniscriptum.com

Printed at: see last page
ISBN: 978-620-8-58525-9

SUMMARY

To my parents Neuza and Antônio, for their constant love, words of comfort, strength and for believing in me.

To Felipe, for understanding my absence as a construction of the future.

To my love Adriano, for being by my side, for believing in my dreams and encouraging me with his love.

To Creusa, for her trust, affection, help and our long conversations.

ACKNOWLEDGMENTS

To the subject Ma., for the affectionate coexistence, for the collaboration, for teaching me so much.

To CNPQ, for their financial support so that this research could be carried out.

To my family (grandparents, aunts, cousins) who understood my absence and always supported me.

My sisters, for understanding and encouraging me, each in their own way, often without understanding why I traveled so much.

To our friends in Maringa who prayed and cheered us on to victory.

My teachers Ana Paula, Carla and Fabiana, exemplary professionals who gave me my foundation and will always be my mirrors.

To the participants in the aphasics group who made me grow as a speech therapist and also as a person.

The speech therapy undergraduates for being present and taking part in my teaching internship.

INTRODUCTION

This researcher's interest in questions about aphasia and its repercussions on language arose during her undergraduate studies when, as an intern, she accompanied a group of aphasics called GOIA (Grupo de Orientaçâo e Integraçâo dos Afâsicos) at the Centro Universitàrio de Maringâ.

These follow-ups gave rise to concerns about the care of aphasics, especially in relation to understanding how their language works, the limitations and specificities resulting from aphasia, especially with issues related to written language.

From the late 1980s onwards, linguists in Brazil have been working on issues related to the linguistic-discursive processes involved in cases of aphasia. Among these studies, we highlight the pioneering work of Coudry, who introduced neurolinguistic studies to the Institute of Language Studies at UNICAMP. This researcher criticizes the evaluation of language carried out and exercised on the domain of the normative written tradition, separated from the intersubjective and social exercise of language.

Based on Santana and Macedo (2006), who argue that studies on aphasia show that the ability to write does not disappear after brain damage, but remains altered, we reaffirm the importance research that provides speech therapists with theoretical arguments capable of outlining conceptions around the aphasic subject and the therapeutic process.

The main aim of this book is to carry out a longitudinal analysis of the language therapy process of an aphasic subject called Ma, considering issues of literacy as a guiding principle.

It should be clarified that, in this research project, literacy is understood, according to Signorini (2001), as a set of social communication practices related to the use of written materials, and which involve actions of a physical, mental and linguistic-discursive nature, as well as social and political-ideological ones.

When considering the importance of literacy in therapeutic work with aphasics, and assuming a discursive conception of language, the therapist moves away from speech therapy practices based on repetition and the complementation of sentences and words. In this way, he seeks to move closer to a meaningful practice with language, recognizing the aphasic as the subject of language, as proposed by Santana and Macedo (2006).

Supported by a conception that sees language as a constitutive activity, the hypothesis is that, by considering the social practice of reading and writing of the aphasic subject, writing is no longer seen as an individual process. This breaks down certain stigmas and (re)inserts the subject, now aphasic, equally into routines that are meaningful to them.

By defending this differentiated proposal, in which orality and writing are seen as interdependent language modalities, the resources offered in the therapeutic process with aphasic subjects are expanded, enabling the speech therapist to go beyond a restrictive vision, focused only on improving speech. In the opposite direction, this perspective, based on an approach that sees language as a social and historical work, shows the speech therapist a possibility of interacting with aphasic subjects that goes beyond exercises based on words and phrases isolated from a meaningful context.

Coudry (1986) argues that therapeutic work with aphasic patients should be carried out in the light of the effective use of language, because it is in language that the subject will re-establish interpersonal and factual relationships and reconstitute himself as a subject differentiated by these relationships and vice versa. Through a dialogic interaction, the aphasic subject begins to assume their role between dialogic turns. According to this author, in the course of expressive resources, language is reconstituted, meaning is negotiated and the dialogical game allows the subject to deal with various facets of the linguistic object, adapting and reflecting on the organization of textual productions.

In defending this hypothesis, some questions arise that motivate the researcher to problematize writing in this study:

- How should therapy be designed when the speech therapist considers the social practices of reading and writing of the aphasic subject?
- What is the role of the speech therapist in a therapeutic process based on meaningful language practices?

In order to answer these questions, the research is organized into five chapters. The first, called Aphasia and Literacy, provides a short historical survey of aphasia and its relationship with written language, drawing a parallel with questions about literacy, the concept of discursive genres and the relationship between orality and writing.

The next chapter, entitled Assessment, Diagnosis and Therapy, describes how the therapeutic process is carried out within the framework of cognitive neuropsychology and neurolinguistics enunciative-discursive.

In the third chapter, we describe the methodological procedures carried out in order to fulfill the proposed objective of the research work. The fourth chapter presents an analysis of Ma's therapeutic process. The fifth and final chapter considers the issues raised.

1 APHASIA AND LITERACY

1.1 WRITTEN LANGUAGE STUDIES IN APHASIA

Interest in the brain/language relationship dates back to ancient times, when Egyptian priests tried to establish anatomical and clinical relationships in sick individuals who were dying. But it wasn't until the 19th century that interest in studying and unraveling the relationship between the brain and language was linked to establishing the cortical localization of language and tackling the question of which parts of the cerebral cortex correspond to different levels of language, both to affirm the localizationist position and to deny it (COUDRY, 1986).

Joseph GALL[1] , in 1806, was the pioneer in establishing the relationship between the damaged central area and the clinical, anatomical and physiological manifestations of impressions seen by the naked eye in the cranial box. And he introduced language among the mental faculties located in the brain (NOPPEY; WALLESH, 2000).

GALL related speech to a certain area of the brain, in a description he called patients with two-speech disorders. He postulated the existence of an organ for words and language in the anterior portion of the brain (frontal lobe). In 1825, Bouillad gathered clinical and pathological evidence to support the GALL hypothesis. In a study of 850 cases, he found lesions in the frontal lobe of 116 patients with speech impairment and insisted on the need to distinguish between two different phenomena in the act of speaking: the power to create words (internal speech) as a sign of our ideas and the power to articulate these same words (external speech). Based on these concepts, Bouillaud suggested that there were two causes that could lead to the loss of speech, each in its own way: one would be the destruction of the word memory organ, and the other, a deficiency in the nervous principle that directs the movements of speech (MUDOCH, 1997).

In 1867, Ogle introduced the term Agraphia to refer to acquired writing disorders as a result of brain damage. In 1881, Exner proposed the existence of a writing center located at the base of the 2nd frontal circumvolution, referring to the motor area of the hand (ARDILA, 2006).

In 1885, Charcot founded what became known as the extreme associationist school. For him, aphasia could be classified into the following forms: verbal blindness, verbal deafness,

1 Gal studied medicine in Vienna and became a renowned neuroanatomist and physiologist. He was a pioneer in the study of the localization of mental functions in the brain. Around 1800 he developed "cranioscopy", a method for guessing personality and the development of mental and moral faculties based on the external shape of the skull. Cranioscopy (*cranium* = skull, *scopos* = vision) was later renamed *phrenology* (*phrenos* = mind, *logos* = study) by his followers.

aphaemia and agraphia. Among these, agraphia, taken according to the author as an alteration linked to written language, would be the consequence of the suspension of a special memory that would allow words to be represented through writing (JAKUBOVICZ; MEINBERG, 1985).

In 1891, Dejérinè described the Alexia syndrome with agraphia. In 1940, Gerstmann proposed that agraphia together with acalculia, right-left disorientation and digital agnosia could appear simultaneously in the same syndrome. Over the next century, different attempts were made to classify agraphia. Goldstein (1948) distinguished two main types of agraphia: apraxic-amnesic and aphasic-amnesic. Lûria (1984) referred to five different groups, three of them associated with aphasic disorders (sensory agraphia, afferent motor agraphia and kinetic motor agraphia) and two resulting from visual-spatial alterations. Hécaen and Albert (1978) distinguished four varieties of agraphia: pure, apraxic, spatial and aphasic. Recently, linguistic classifications have been proposed, which include phonological, lexical and deep agraphia (ARDILA, 2006).

For the authors, these terminologies are directly related to the clinical method of classification, which consists of comparing anatomical findings and correlating them with the linguistic symptoms observed. Each of the symptoms and behaviors is described by the authors as a semiological item.

According to Novaes-Pinto and Santana (2009), the "*inventory of these semiological items or symptoms, organized or recategorized into syndromes, reflects the conditions of production of knowledge and beliefs in a given society*". (p. 20). For the authors, the concern with terminology in the medical sciences stems from the need to develop a "*technical jargon*" that would serve to exchange information between doctors and patients.

From a semiological point of view, aphasia is generally discussed from four aspects: oral expression, written expression, oral comprehension and written comprehension (NOVAES-PINTO E SANTANA, 2009).

If semiology is directly related to diagnosis, tests play a mediating role in this process. However, in the search for answers, for conceptual determinations, for names, the functions are lost. Theoretical presuppositions claim to be concerned with a social characterization with the pattern of the lesion, the insertion and the history of the subject, and end up reducing the aspects assessed to names based on decontextualized metalinguistic functions. It is believed within discursive neurolinguistics that through a contextualized activity, which seeks to carry out the discursive activity of written language in a conscious way, it is possible to understand the aphasic subject's ability to deal with written language (comprehension and production) without reducing it to a merely testing activity.

In Coudry's (1986) definition, aphasia is currently considered to be a disorder characterized by alterations in linguistic processes of meaning of articulatory and discursive origin, produced by focal lesions acquired in the central nervous system. These lesions, located in cortical and/or subcortical areas, may or may not be associated with cognitive damage. The author considers that a subject becomes aphasic when, from a linguistic point of view, the functioning of their language lacks certain production and interpretation resources.

Gil (2003) states that aphasias are language disorders that can affect both expression and reception, including writing, due to specific brain lesions that compromise language areas. In other words, it can be said that studies of aphasia serve as hypotheses for the processing of written language.

Since the last few decades of the last century, the way of thinking about reading and writing has changed enormously. Scholars in the fields of education, speech therapy and others have changed their views on language and it is now seen as a dynamic process that makes up significant contexts of social activity in all its aspects, be they family, community, professional or religious. In addition, it is understood that a person does not learn solely from what is individual, but from the context that surrounds them, including discourses produced in their networks of social relationships.

In order to better understand these transformations in the understanding of language that have been taking place on the part of different professionals, it is important to define and analyze questions about "Literacy".

1.2 LITERACY AND DISCURSIVE GENRES

The term *literacy* comes from the English word *liter. Literacy* comes from the Latin *Littera* which means letter, plus the suffix *cy* which denotes quality, condition, state, fact of being. *Literacy* is therefore the state or condition assumed by those who learn to read and write (SOARES, 2003).

Soares (2003) defines literacy as: *"the state or condition of individuals or social groups in literate societies who effectively exercise the social practices of reading and writing (...)",* i.e. a social phenomenon. When considering literacy, the focus shifts to ways of conceiving reading and writing. It seeks to understand what the subject does, why they do it and what they do when they use the written word. For Infante (2000), the importance that writing assumes for individuals is closely related to the uses, values and functions attributed to this language modality by the societies in which it is inserted.

The concept of Literacy emerged as a way of explaining the impact of writing in all spheres of social activity and not just in school activities, since this concept was created to refer to the uses of written language in the most varied social situations.

To understand the process of literacy, according to Mey (2001), is to understand how subjects act with and on social discourses, and how they use *their own voices*. These voices described would be the social discourses constituting our own discourses.

From this perspective, it is possible to have people who are illiterate or have a rudimentary level of literacy and who are literate. Even if someone doesn't master the written code, it's practically impossible not to know at least one literacy event and participate in some kind of literacy practice, according to the social context in which they are inserted.

Thus, "literate" refers to the possibility of productively handling, in the midst of specific social practices, materials that contain writing, regardless of the degree or level of literacy (FREIRE, 2005).

It is thus understood that literacy studies are not restricted only to people who have acquired writing skills, i.e. those who are literate. Rather, these studies also investigate the consequences of the absence of writing at an individual level, but always referring to the wider social context, i.e. looking, among other things, to see which characteristics of the social structure link the subject with language.

In literate societies, the importance of writing in people's lives is widespread and significant, not only in reading and writing activities themselves, but also in oral activities, since the speech of literate people is very much marked by written language. Writing has become indispensable, that is, its practice and social evaluation have elevated it to a higher status, coming to symbolize education, development and power.

Literacy emerged as a way of explaining the impact of writing on all spheres of human activity and not just school activities, as it is a concept created to refer to the uses of written language everywhere, in everyday life. This has broadened the view of literacy and changed the concept of illiteracy, realizing that literacy goes beyond the act of reading and writing, and refers to the use that each individual makes of reading and writing socially.

The absence as much as the presence of writing in a society are important factors that act both as a cause and a consequence of social, cultural and psychological transformations that are sometimes radical.

Analyzing the written language of aphasics from this theoretical position allows the therapist to stop seeing writing as something that is individually constituted. This position, according to Santana and Macedo (2006), takes into account the literacy practices that the aphasic subject has been involved in since before becoming aphasic. These practices are fundamental for their (re)insertion into reading and writing activities. Understanding the link that the aphasic subject had with written language and the social importance attributed to it before the aphasia allows the speech therapist to organize their actions towards the subject in their relationship with language (SANTANA, 2002).

The written texts produced by aphasics reveal their participation in interlocutive situations. The constitution of meaning takes place in oral and written dialogic situations and in these situations it is possible to follow the different ways in which the aphasic places themselves as a subject in the interaction. Even if there is an initial denial on the part of the aphasic subject in relation to the ability to use reading and writing, this denial can be minimized precisely because of this subject's need to participate in the interactive process. This need can be seen in the textual insertions made by the subjects, to the extent that their interlocutor invites them to take part in this process by taking an interest in understanding what they are writing. This is how some risk writing even "without thinking they can".

Speech and writing seen as products of social practices determine the place, role and degree of relevance of orality and literacy practices in a society, justifying the positioning of the relationship between them on the axis of a socio-historical continuum.

This socio-historical continuum of oral and written practices, in the case of aphasics, allows the therapist to value and understand the particular mechanisms that each subject uses to interact with others, even after the difficulties related to the neurological episode (CÔRREA, 2004).

With regard to the differences between oral and written practices, it should be emphasized, according to Marcuschi (2001), that they occur within a *typological continuum* of social practices of textual production and not in the dichotomous relationship of two opposing poles. In this sense, correlations are established on various levels, resulting in "a set of variations". This fact is exemplified by Marcuschi in the following figure:

Figure 1 - SPEECH AND WRITING IN THE CONTINUUM OF TEXTUAL GENRES

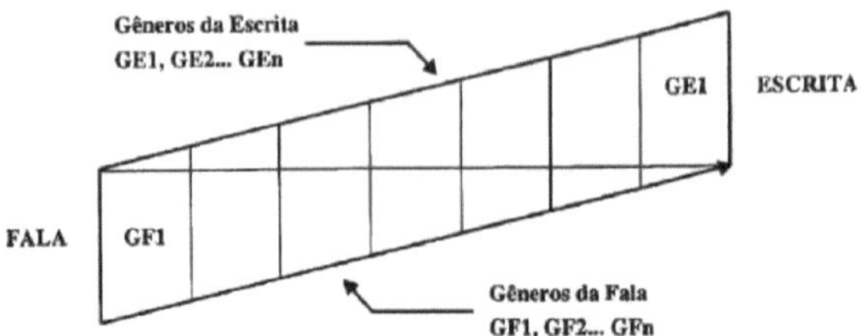

SOURCE: MARCUSCHI, 2001b, p.38 58

It is clear from the picture above that speaking and writing take place on two continuums:

a) The continuum of textual genres (GF1, GF2....GFn and GEI, GE2.... GEn);

b) The continuum of speech and writing characteristics.

Different types of texts are produced in the most varied domains of discourse, both oral and written. The figure above shows how these texts intersect at certain times, forming mixed language domains in these situations. As an example of this,

Marcuschi cites television news texts: these are originally written texts, received by the "reader" orally. It follows, then, that orality and writing cannot be situated in different linguistic systems, because they are both part of the same language system. Not as a form of representation of each other, but as a blend of the oral and written modalities of language.

To explain this blending, i.e. the mixed relationships of textual genres, Marcuschi starts from relationships between media and conceptions, with speech being an oral concept and a sound medium, and writing, a written concept and a graphic medium. The author represents the mixed domains in the figure below.

FIGURE 2 - REPRESENTATION OF ORALITY AND WRITING BY MEANS OF PRODUCTION AND DISCURSIVE CONCEPTION

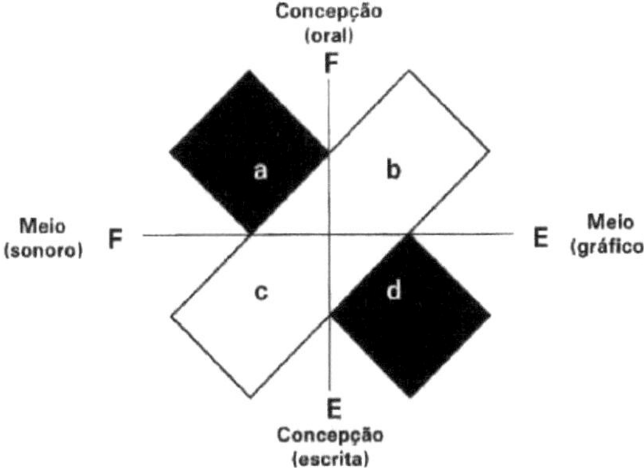

SOURCE: MARCUSCHI, 2001b, p.38

Thus, for Marcuschi, "a" is the domain of the typically *spoken (orality)*, both in terms of medium and concept, and the counterpart "d" corresponds to the *written* domain, so "b" and "c" correspond to the mixed domains, and this would be the "place" where the mixtures of speech and writing (as the two forms of language representation) occur.

In this way, the relationship between speech and writing, seen as a *continuum* of social practices, distances itself from strict dichotomies. With this, it is assumed that both speech and writing vary, and their relationships should be analyzed as two modalities of language use, taking language as a constitutive activity of the subject.

In aphasia, according to Garcez (1998), this relationship between orality and writing has peculiar characteristics, since each of these practices can play different roles during an interaction situation. These are mechanisms such as gestures, drawings, writing in the air, among others, which aphasics use to make themselves understood.

According to Macedo (2006), this transit between orality and writing gives the subjects a *continuum* between these modalities, because in many moments, for example, writing replaces speech, and in the next moment it mediates the interlocutive relationship itself. Furthermore, according to the author, the joint construction of texts produced by aphasics occurs in such a way that these subjects also move between orality and writing in an attempt to maintain the interlocutive process.

For Marchuschi (2001), the analysis of the relationship between speech and writing is done within the process of dialogic interaction, and language is understood as an interactive and dynamic phenomenon, focused on the dialogic activities that mark the most salient characteristics of speech. According to Street (1995), this is one of the best ways of observing literacy and orality as social practices.

From this point of view, it is possible to deal with the phenomena of comprehension in face-to-face interaction and in the interaction between the reader and the written text, in order to detect specificities in the very activity of constructing meanings, following a discursive and interpretative line (MARCHUSCHI, 2001).

These concrete situations of social interaction are defined as discursive genres, considered by Bakhtin (1997) as relatively stable types of utterances, which are composed within interactional spheres. According to the author, utterances reflect the specific conditions and purposes of the spheres of human activity, not only through their content and verbal style, but also through their compositional construction. The totality of an utterance is organized, among other factors, by the *discursive intent,* which helps in the choice of the genre to be used at the moment of interaction, since all utterances are part of a genre, which contains a standard and relatively stable way of structuring a whole. Genres organize our speech and vary according to the circumstances of communication, the social position and personal relationship of the interlocutors. Therefore, in order for verbal communication to be effective, one must have knowledge not only of language, but also of the genres of discourse. (BAKHTIN, 1997)

The discursive genre, according to Rojo (2001), has an important bearing on the situations in which the statements are produced in terms of their socio-historical aspects, the conditions of production that are taken into account by the writer depending on the situation and their objectives. The discourse determines what should be said (content), while the genre determines how it should be said (style), based on the context in which it is announced.

For Santana and Macedo (2006), understanding how the aphasic subject deals with discursive genres before the neurological episode and analyzing what this relationship is like after the subject has become aphasic, is to open up a path for the recovery of this new subject who now has aphasia.

In this way, reflection on discursive genres brings the speech therapist face to face with the notion of discourse as an interlocutive process. This notion guides clinical practice with the language of aphasic subjects, taking into account all the emergences of reading and writing acts, such as: reading and writing itself, drawings, writing gestures, writing numbers, leafing through a magazine. This allows the speech therapist to understand that the written language of aphasics only occurs with these particularities because it is inserted in a certain discursive space.

It's worth pointing out that some aphasia sufferers have more difficulties with writing and others with speaking, but the participation of aphasic sufferers in significant situations of use of oral and written language ends up bringing about changes in the subject in relation to writing and language in general.

2 ASSESSMENT, DIAGNOSIS AND THERAPY

The need to intervene on and with the language of aphasic subjects was strengthened in the 20th century, due to the large number of ex-combatants with brain injuries and speech/language problems who survived the great world wars. These wars led society to organize activities for the rehabilitation of the injured, with aphasics occupying a prominent place. An immediate response to the post-war situation was the publication of a vast number of treatises on aphasia and its assessment, which culminated in the publication of a large number of tests in all countries (ORTIZ, 2005).

The post-war preoccupation brought together various researchers on aphasia: neurologists, psychologists, psychiatrists, speech therapists and linguists (FONSECA, 2002). These professionals sought to understand the causes and consequences of the lesions in each individual, trying to propose ways of rehabilitating them. In this way, various theoretical currents emerged to address these issues.

This chapter aims to describe cognitive neuropsychology and enunciative-discursive neurolinguistics. The former is one of the most traditional. According to Kristensen, Almeida and Goes (2001), neuropsychological assessment arose with the aim of seeking correlations between neuroanatomical findings and cognitive failures present in patients with obvious brain damage. Major changes have occurred in its methods, partly as a result of technological advances during the 135 years of neuropsychology's existence.

The importance of describing enunciative-discursive neurolinguistics stems from the fact that it is the approach that will underpin the entire discussion and analysis of the data in this dissertation. Coudry's (1986) work was one of the pioneers in dealing with enunciative-discursive neurolinguistics, taking on a perspective in working with and through language that includes the subject, rather than a theorization focused solely on the symptom and what is missing in their speech/writing.

2.1 COGNITIVE NEUROPSYCHOLOGY

Neuropsychology emerged as a result of studies into the relationship between aphasia and brain damage. Currently, its studies link cognition and human behavior, as well as preserved or altered brain functions (KRISTENSEN, ALMEIDA, GOMES, 2001).

Initially, the anatomical-clinical correlation was based on clinical observations of unique cases compared with the results of *post-mortem* anatomical analyses. There is no doubt that two world wars brought about a great advance in neuropsychological assessment. Techniques emerged that allowed neural functioning to be investigated.

The great wars were also responsible for the participation of psychologists in the study of the relationship between the brain and cognitive functions due to the large population of trauma patients, involving a greater number of professionals interested in assessing neuropsychological recovery work. Psychology has contributed to the development of neuropsychology in three ways: (1) improving methods of assessing cognitive functions, (2) presenting theoretical bases on cognition and the notion of cognitive processes and their breakdowns and (3) methods of recovering patients with cognitive difficulties resulting from brain injuries (KRISTENSEN, ALMEIDA E GOMES, 2001).

The main body of neuropsychological knowledge derives from the study of neurological patients with brain lesions with a known and circumscribed location. From studies of such patients, a large number of psychological tests were developed. These emphasized the study of cognitive processes (mental functions) rather than performance on performance tests or the location of the lesion. Psychological tests are used to try to identify, as precisely as possible, the cognitive processes that are impaired in a patient with brain damage.

According to Parente (1997), rehabilitation work for aphasics should begin with a thorough assessment. To do this, some aspects must be considered, such as

- The examiner's view of a particular test;
- The data received from the neurological examination, such as etiology, size and location of the lesion and neuropsychological data;
- Individual patient data relevant to the theory of brain organization for language and data on socio-cultural level and personality that may be interfering with the performance of the assessment;
- Data related to the therapy, i.e. data that considers the therapy as a continuum of the evaluation carried out.

According to Antonio (2004), neuropsychological assessment is based on the dynamic localization of functions, with the aim of investigating higher cortical functions such as attention, memory, language and perception, among others. This assessment is structured in such a way as to explore the functional integrity of the brain, demonstrated through the level of development manifested by behavior.

Far from a localized view of brain functions, neuropsychology understands the participation of the brain as a whole in which the areas are interdependent and interrelated, functioning like an orchestra, which depends on the integration of its components to perform a concert. Proposed by Luria (1984), this integration of brain areas was called a functional system.

In this direction, cognitive neuropsychology uses specifically standardized tests to assess neuropsychological functions, mainly involving attention, perception, language, reasoning, abstraction, memory, learning, academic skills, information processing, visual construction, affect, motor and executive functions (ANTUNHA, 2002).

The results of these scales and tests reflect the main gains throughout development and aim to determine the specific evolutionary level. The importance of these tools, according to neuropsychologists, lies mainly in the prevention and early detection of developmental/learning disorders, indicating in detail the pace and quality of the process and enabling a qualitative and quantitative "mapping" of the brain areas and their interconnections (functional system), with a view to early and precise therapeutic interventions. Far beyond the simple administration of tests, the quantitative results reflect the conceptual maturity and cognitive level of these patients, while the qualitative results express the main gains and potential (ANDRADE, 2004).

For cognitive neuropsychology, therapeutic interventions, according to Parente (1997), should focus on re-establishing information in memory or reorganizing procedures, i.e. accessing the memory of literal representations again, even if by other mechanisms. In order to achieve an effective treatment result, certain points must be taken into account when formulating strategies: verbal and non-verbal intelligence, schooling, practical and occupational life habits, interests and motivations of the subjects.

The aim is to get the subject to access the memory of the Iteral representations again, albeit by other mechanisms, in other words, to try to "recover" the damaged route.

Within this neuropsychological approach, Parente (1997) defines the role of the speech therapist as broadly investigating aphasic manifestations, as well as the interrelationship between them, considering language processing models and the sub-processes that occur in each specific activity.

For the author, only with this vision will the professional be able to carry out an appropriate therapeutic intervention, aiming to improve functions and maximize available resources, through compensatory strategies.

Analyzing the data using compensatory tasks will allow the speech therapist, according to the neuropsychological approach, to carry out appropriate therapy planning, including taking into account favorable or unfavorable points in terms of rehabilitation prognosis, allowing the subject's care to be shorter and more effective.

In order to rehabilitate writing within cognitive neuropsychology, it is first necessary to understand the nature of the disorder by understanding which processes necessary for writing are failing or maintained within the Functional Architecture (CARTHERY & PARENTE, 2006).

Helping the subject to make full use of all residual written and oral skills, using auditory stimulation to elicit language, is the basic principle of aphasic rehabilitation, according to Ortiz (2005). It is up to the therapist, according to this perspective, to choose the right stimulus for the subject, so that it has meaning for the patient.

According to Salles (2001), Cognitive Neuropsychology allied to the cognitive models of normal reading and impaired reading proposed by Cognitive Psychology, Information Processing Theory, leads to a better understanding of neurological damage, and consequently to the development of strategies for speech therapy intervention.

Successful intervention within neuropsychology requires a careful, multidimensional assessment. The process of assessing cognitive/linguistic factors must be closely linked to theoretical models of learning to read/write. The way in which the assessment is carried out depends on which factors are considered central to the cognitive system (PINHEIRO, 1995).

Until about 30 years ago, the main objective of neuropsychology was to establish a correlation between brain structure and mental operations. A period in which the therapist was responsible for assessing the patient's symptoms and indicating the location of the lesion. Currently, neuropsychological rehabilitation is dedicated to training altered cognitive processes, which are assessed by tests, to reduce attention disorders, language, visual processing, memory, reasoning, problem solving and executive functions (planning, organization, etc.). The exercises are aimed at clinical restoration or compensation of functions.

The view of language that underpins all cognitive neuropsychology therapy is a strictly classical one. Language is conceived as a code, as a structure or a system of pre-established rules.

In contrast to this approach, enunciative-discursive neurolinguistics has a view of language that focuses on the subject and their potential, considering that subjects are social authors. They are active, and dialogically constitute and are constituted in socio-verbal interaction.

2.2 ENUNCIATIVE-DISCURSIVE NEUROLINGUISTICS

Discursive Neurolinguistics is made up of a set of theories and practices whose conception of language, contrary to an organicist view, conceives of language, discourse, brain and mind as human characteristics that are related. In this direction, the hypothesis of historicity and the indeterminacy of language are, in particular, conceived as the work and creative force of language itself and of each subject, according to Franchi (1977/1992).

Neurolinguistic studies that follow the discursive tradition develop a form of linguistic-cognitive evaluation based on discursive practices (Maingueneau, 1989). These practices make sense to people who are part of the society in which we live, evidenced in some way in collective and individual sessions, above all through the social use of speech, writing and reading.

In the specific case of aphasic people, they are seen as producers of discourse, inserted in social practices and producers of processes of meaning. The interest here is not in aphasia as an unstructured language, but in the aphasic, in their social reintegration.

Alternative processes of signification, according to Coudry (1986), are resources that the aphasic uses to act as a speaker through language, the body/gestures and perception. These processes take place in the interlocution that takes place between the aphasic and the non-aphasic, the meaning of which is not pre-determined, but is made in the midst of a series of anthropo-cultural factors that qualify the interaction in question.

In order to understand the processes of meaning that occur in the language of the aphasic subject, it is necessary to relate the processes of discovery and knowledge of the difficulties that the subject presents, as well as the alternative processes of meaning that he uses to deal with them. In other words, we need to understand what the subject's language is like and how it occurs in different discursive situations (COUDRY, 1986).

The language of the aphasic subject is always incomplete in relation to what they want to say (Freud, 1969), which is put into words (involving the body, gestures, perceptions, associations, facial expressions) in what is said by one and understood by the other. In interlocution, the most varied conditions in which saying/doing/showing takes place are faced.

The subject, as Franchi (1977/1992) argues, works linguistically to produce meanings; and aphasic subjects also do this. Conceiving language apart from its functioning and from the subject who enunciates it is the preferred path of traditional studies, which differ radically from those assumed by Discursive Neurolinguistics. In this context, a new reading of the pathological phenomena of language is possible, seeking to understand, on the one hand, the difficulties that the aphasic manifests in the use of language and, on the other, the alternative processes of signification that the aphasic practices as a solution to face them (Coudry, 1986).

Since subjects are different from each other, the language of aphasic subjects is also subject to this difference. This is why some aphasics speak more and others less, and thus play the role of language subject. In order to effectively assess these subjects within this approach, Coudry (1986) states that it is necessary to consider that the aphasic is inserted in a linguistic and cultural community, and that they produce meaningful activities for the clinician and the aphasic to act with and on language. In this way, Coudry proposes activities such as: personal life stories, showing photos, commenting on news events, reading and discussing newspapers, magazines, news reports, making diaries and so on.

According to Arantes (2005), the speech therapist who works with aphasic subjects, in their clinical practice, is confronted precisely with the face of language that escapes the rule, with what is not predictable, with what is residual. In the clinic, the linguistic phenomenon reveals its most inapprehensible and heterogeneous face. Language in its pathological dimension is the clearest and greatest expression of the singular, the individual. It is the revelation of a singularity inscribed in language.

During the assessment and therapeutic process, according to Zambioni (2007), the speech therapist must pay attention to the moments of interlocution between therapist and aphasic subject. It is also important to pay attention to the circumstances of non-word that are part of the verbal activity of these subjects, since all these moments are part of the alternative processes used by aphasics.

It is understood from discursive neurolinguistics that the evaluative and therapeutic process must be a continuum in the midst of contextualized interactive episodes, so that linguistic processes are (re)constructed and (re)organized.

For Santana (2002), in an efficient therapeutic process, writing must be analyzed as a social activity. This form of language should be considered as an integral part of the subject's journey, being understood as a privileged place for the manifestation of the subject's uniqueness.

Working with written language with aphasics from this discursive enunciative perspective is still under-researched. Despite an extensive bibliographic survey of scientific journals and search engines, it was only possible to identify the authors Santana (2002) and Macedo (2006) as researchers involved with this topic. As Macedo reports, traditionally, studies on aphasia have sought to identify difficulties with written language resulting from brain damage in the same way that alterations in oral language are identified. These studies are based on a perspective that takes language and the subject from a reductionist point of view.

Santana (2002) surveys the view of written language in aphasiology, analyzing its history up to current neuropsychological research, stressing that aphasics are part of a literate society. For her, it is important to see how the characteristics of this society reflect on the subject's relationship with their writing. And it is up to the speech therapist to take a discursive stance towards written language, trying to understand how it works and considering writing as a *discursive praxis*, and this is only possible, according to the author, through an exercise in subjectivity, dialogism and linguistic work.

According to Macedo (2006), written language activities developed by aphasic individuals are produced more fluently through collaborative interlocution with another person, preferably a writer. The situational context and the conditions of production (enunciative, interactive conditions between aphasic subjects and their interlocutors) are part of the enunciative event in which rephrasing takes place. The literacy processes of the writing subjects are constitutive of the written textual reworkings produced by the aphasic subjects. Macedo states that it is fundamental, in this process, to consider the conditions of literacy, the situations of interaction during the production of the written text and the possibilities for aphasic subjects to rephrase in these contexts.

Santana and Macedo's (2006) proposal has as its main goal the use of writing in the subjects' daily lives, not just its formal use. Within this enunciative-discursive vision defended by the authors, therapeutic work must try to transform the relationship of suffering that this subject establishes in the face of their current condition with language. A focus on literacy allows speech therapists to assume the privileged position of mediators and interlocutors of these subjects within the therapeutic space, trying to favor situations in which the social practices of reading and writing are established.

For Santana (2002), the therapist must be a privileged interlocutor, who knows the linguistic processes of reading and writing, so that they can propose therapeutic strategies aimed at (re)inserting the subject into language. Macedo (2006) states that "*the speech therapist must focus on recovering the possibility of signifying the world and being signified by it*"

In order for the speech therapist to achieve results in the therapeutic process and to be able to act as an interlocutor, it is necessary to have a theoretical knowledge of discursive issues, from which Language is understood as an interlocutive process and as constitutive work.

After describing the two approaches, it becomes clear that the notion of meaning in aphasic speech is given in the use of language as a defined activity, and that the differences between speech and writing must be seen and analyzed from the perspective of "use" and not from that of the "system". Thus, the relationships between the two forms of language modality will also be centered on the "uses of linguistic codes".

For these reasons, this research moves away from theoretical models and strict dichotomies as set out in the first part of this chapter, in order to discard standard tests and decontextualized clinical practice, and starts to adopt an assessment and monitoring centered on discursive conditions, in order to incorporate the appropriate concepts of language as interaction.

3 METHODOLOGICAL PROCEDURES

This chapter will describe the methodological procedures used in this research. However, before describing the details of the research itself, it is important to understand specifically what research is. Research involves systematic, critical and self-critical investigation with the aim of contributing to the advancement of knowledge (BASSEY, 1990).

Research is systematic because the collection and analysis of data is supported by reason or theory. It is critical because the data collected must be subject to careful examination by the researcher in order to ensure that it is valuable and represents what is intended. It is self-critical because researchers are expected to use self-criticism in the decisions they make about the research. (MOREIRA and CALEFFE, 2006)

For Bagno (2003), the richness of research lies in the research itself, in the process of investigation, in the exploration of the material, in the application of theories, in the raising of hypotheses. It is the research itself, the very process of investigation that is important, and not always just the product of the work. Research is much richer if, instead of a few answers, it proposes new questions, new problems, new incentives to do more research. Research cannot be viewed in a mechanical, bureaucratic way.

The theme of this research is Literacy and Aphasia, with the general objective of analyzing the therapeutic process of an aphasic subject. The production of linguistic data took place in interactive situations of conversation, reading and writing during speech therapy sessions, involving therapist and aphasic subject. The case study was chosen because the practice is centered on a discursive line established through interactive and dialogical situations. In this way, historical and cultural issues were included in the case which, in a constant and continuous way, portray the subject/language relationship which the statistical perspective does not take into account. The data analysis corresponds to a longitudinal follow-up of the case, which allows us to highlight the growth in the reconstruction of the subject's language.

The choice of methodology is primarily due to the concept of language on which this research is based. This means that the reduced notion of language as a communication code has been discarded, as well as the hypothesis of language as a faculty of the human mind, as these ideas restrict the description of aphasia to linguistic deficits. In opposition to this thinking, we adopt a conception of language that is in line with that proposed by Franchi (1977), observing the assumption that language is a constitutive activity. This concept is also developed by Coudry, who states that language "*integrates its functioning in the contextual and social dimension in which men, through it, act on others, in the subjective dimension in which, through it, men constitute themselves as subjects, in the cognitive dimension in which, through it, men act on the world by structuring reality*" (COUDRY, 1986, p.47).

In this way, data collection moves away from classic linguistic practices, which are centered on standardized tests, and uses metalinguistic activities. Another reason that justifies this methodological choice is the possibility it offers of demonstrating, by analyzing the data of an aphasic subject, the relationship established between orality and writing, as he seeks to restructure his language when inserted into interactive situations.

The episodes in this study were collected during speech therapy sessions, which were recorded on both cassette and video tapes. Writing data was collected at the same time as oral data, because of its occurrence. The writing productions that the aphasic subject brought from home were also dated and attached to the writing data collected in the recorded therapy sessions. The importance of recording the sessions was discussed with Ma, who understood, agreed and authorized the recording, use and publication of the data in this research.

The data collection period lasted from March 2008 until the end of July 2009. The therapy sessions were interrupted during school vacations. The location of the recordings was always the speech therapy room, and each session lasted between 40 and 50 minutes. The therapist, following the linguistic-discursive line, not only positioned herself as an interlocutor in the dialogic situations, but also as a mediator, with a view to helping the aphasic to recognize his role in the interlocution, differentiating himself from the interlocutor-investigator, and to work on his linguistic difficulties.

The convention established to identify the interlocutors in the transcription of the data is as follows: Ig for therapist and Ma for the aphasic subject. It should be emphasized that at no time during the recording sessions was there any other interlocutor than the two specified here. The discursive situations analyzed are divided into episodes that follow an ordinal numbering from 1 to 8. The data was chosen by the therapist with a view to different discursive genres and an evolution of both the therapeutic process and Ma's relationship with her language and with the therapist (Ig).

3.1 PARTICIPATING SUBJECT

One aphasic subject, identified as Ma. Male, 45 years old.

The subject will be presented in more detail at the beginning of Chapter 4.

3.2 LOCAL

The research took place on the premises of the Speech Therapy Clinic of the Tuiuti University of Paranà, located in the city of Curitiba.

4 DATA ANALYSIS

4.1 SUBJECT MA

Ma is a 45-year-old man, divorced, the father of two daughters (one aged 27 and the other 23) and the grandfather of two granddaughters (one aged 6 and the other 3). He has a high school education. He was a driver and traveled to various places in Brazil.

On June 16, 2006, Ma was driving a friend home. Late at night, he stopped at a traffic light and was mugged. After that, he said he didn't remember anything, only when he woke up in hospital. According to the medical records, Ma was the victim of a "beating" to the skull. CT scans indicated a left temporoparietal traumatic brain injury and hemorrhage in the underlying parenchyma. He was referred by his neurologist on 06/03/07 for speech therapy, as he had a sequelae of TBI (traumatic brain injury).

He currently lives alone at the back of his sister's house and carries out all his daily activities independently. His routine is to walk in the Botanical Garden and do some household chores, such as cleaning the house, cooking, washing the sidewalk, among others. She likes going for walks, shopping and traveling.

He reported that right after the accident he didn't speak at all, just stared at people.

Speech therapy began on April 9, 2008. In this first interview, Ma said that he was feeling better, that he could now count money, drive and travel by car to other places outside of Curitiba. He is sometimes annoyed by strangers who think he is a foreigner because of his speech difficulties. According to him, he would like them to know about his problem.

In this first meeting, we tried to understand Ma's main complaints and also to begin the process of understanding his relationship with language.

The main complaint was related to resuming writing, as Ma wanted to renew her driver's license (as shown in the transcript below).

DATE: 09/04/08

[1] Ig: (...) Do you think that after the accident your reading and writing were impaired?

[2] Ma: It's hard for me to say. Before I didn't know anything, now ... ((*took a piece of paper and began to* [3] *write 1, 2, 3 ...*))

[4] Ig: What's it like for ler?

[5] Ma: It's hard to say...

[6] Ig: But can you understand what you read?

Ma: ((*Affirmative gesture with her head*)) Needs to improve oh ... 2 ((*shows the wallet of driver*))
Ig: Are you going to renew your driver's license? Ah! Two years from now, there's still time (...)

That day, he tried to show how much he had improved and that he was able to write in sequence (alphabet and numbers). He also said that his daughter, who is a teacher, had helped him by giving him some exercises to copy.

The data collected on his reading and writing habits revealed that, before the accident, Ma didn't read very often, just a few articles. As for his writing habits, he said that he used this language modality in his routine when he signed checks, filled out invoices, among other things.

Even though orality is significantly more used by the majority of society, written characteristics are strongly intertwined with orality in a graphocentric society like ours. Of course, Ma's reading and writing skills are much broader and so is his use of them, which is why I used literacy as the guiding principle in this research.

Figure 3 Date: 09/04/08

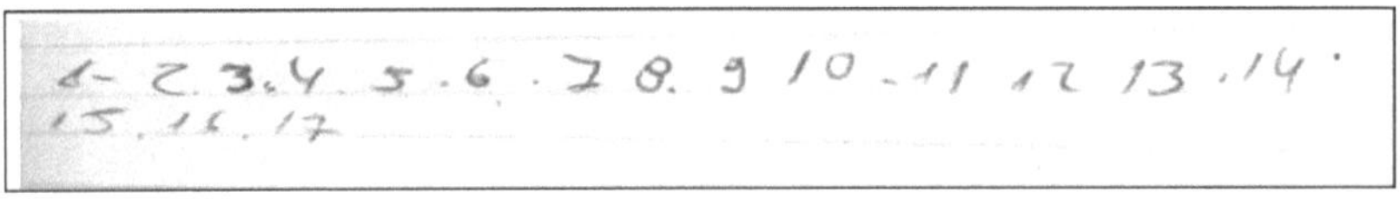

1- 2.3.4 5.6.7 8. 9 10.11 12 13.14.
15.16.17

The first impression gained from this initial interview is related to the anxiety Ma generated when she had to use orality. The main point was her difficulty in naming: first names, street names and common names necessary for the construction of an account of her routine. If the therapist were based on standardized cognitive neuropsychology tests, her vision would be restricted to the difficulties present in the subject's orality.

However, based on an enunciative-discursive vision, the therapist tried to focus on the resources he used to interact. It was possible to see the resources he used: gestures, drawings and his own writing.

Figure 3 shows Ma's writing of numbers. As he scribbled on the paper, he said that he knew how to write and that he had improved a little since his accident. This demonstrated Ma's conflict over his language after the neurological episode, and was also exemplified when he repeated several times the statement: "I knew, now I don't know anymore".

For Ma, writing this sequence of numbers is of great importance, because as he himself says: "*he can still write",* it's related to the way he deals with his aphasia. In everyday life, the formal use of this sequence of numbers becomes irrelevant, because it has no specific social function, it is not related to Ma's daily life.

According to Macedo (2004), when aphasics themselves carry out an "analysis" of their writing, they have an ideal form of writing as a yardstick, which leads them to a personal conflict in the face of their own difficulties, especially when they compare their current writing with their writing before aphasia (or with their idea of writing before aphasia).

1. Episode (09/04/08)

In order to get to know Ma, the first sessions focused on his life story. Starting with family photographs and personal accounts, discursive work began with Ma who, as he told stories about himself or his family, the "ice" was broken and the bond with Ig increased with each session, which allowed the work of reworking the altered language.

Ma liked to tell stories about his life; being a truck driver, he traveled a lot and had many curious situations to relate, such as: giving birth in the ambulance; putting out fires, among others. Recounting his life was something he enjoyed very much, as was telling stories about his youth. And as the therapist also went on several trips, she also related some events. Ma was enthusiastic when, after the sessions, he listened to his recorded productions.

Ma uses other mechanisms of signification to deal with the difficulty of lexical access that makes naming difficult in his speech.

From the beginning of the work, Ma used orality and writing concomitantly (as in a process of complementarity between the two) in the situations of dialogic interactions that arose in the therapeutic sessions.

In the data shown below, we can see how Ma makes use of various verbal and non-verbal resources to establish an interaction with the other.

Data 1/orality

[1] L3 Ig: Did you wake up at 5 o'clock?

[2] Ma: No (...)

[3] Ig: 7 hours? And what did you do?

[4] Ma: ((*Wrote on paper 6:30))*

[5] Ig: What did you do when you woke up at 6:30?

[6] Ma: Yeah... I don't know ... before I knew ... ((*gesture of running))*

[7] Ig: CO... CO...

[8] Ma: RUNNING ... There ... near ... every day ((*picks up the map the therapist brought from Curitiba))*

[9] *((shows the Botanical Garden)).*

Data 1 /writing

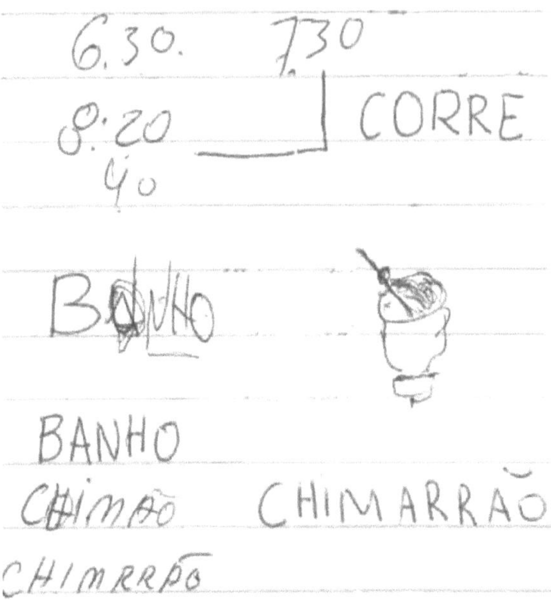

In the episode reported above, we can see that Ma achieves meaning in an intersubjective situation. In addition, as Mayrink-Sabinson (2002, p.121) points out, Ma's productions show the "presence of rephrasing" which "superimposes a 'correction' on writing that has not been erased", as in the writing of "Bunho" and "Chimâo". Orality and writing establish an interrelationship, even in this episode. Ma positions herself as an active subject through oral and written language. She uses writing with the aim of "not writing a text, but speaking a text". In other words, he uses writing as an expressive resource, "the act of writing functions as a support capable of 'providing' him with communication, in which writing itself does not communicate, but only serves as an instrument to trigger oral enunciation" (SANTANA, 2002, p.99). Therefore, the Ma subject "writes to speak" (takes the attitude of writing to achieve meaning in interaction), a more detailed explanation of which can be found in the master's thesis by Luciana C. L. Flosi (2003). L. Flosi (2003), "The Dynamic Relationship of Oral Language with Writing and Gestures in Aphasia", when she describes the two subjects: NF and MG, both use writing, as in the case of subject Ma (described in this research), for orality. The subject NF demonstrates the attitude of writing, while MG starts from drawing, arrives at writing and in this way develops an internalized process of language in order to speak (p.29 to 35). Throughout the session, Ig was signifying the writing and relating it to Ma's speech. As can be seen in the writing data that Ma writes the time and then with the therapist's handwriting, this time is related to the start and end of the activity and Ig also describes in this data what activity he is carrying out. It is up to the speech therapist to go much further than understanding how language works, it is necessary to understand what resources each aphasic uses to interact with others through language. In order to understand these resources, a series of historical factors are taken into account, both for the aphasic and the non-aphasic.

2nd Episode (30/04/08)

The episode that will be analyzed below refers to a situation that occurred during Ma's fourth speech therapy session. As the subject felt more comfortable telling us about the events of his life, Ig asked Ma to bring in photographs, arguing that it would be a good way of getting to know his family and friends and would help him write his biography (work developed in the aphasics group). In this episode, Ma shows the photos in his wallet and tells us a little about his sisters.

Data 2 / orality

[1] Ma: ((takes his driver's license out of his pocket and shows it as it was before))

[2] Ma: I had the business, but I don't have it anymore

[3] Ig: Business? What did you have?

[4] Ma: I had it here ((points to photo and runs hand through hair)) òi here!

[5] Ig: He had hair, right? ((laughs)) New here, huh?

[6] M: But also ... how long?

(...)

[7] Ma: After she leaves. Oh, she ... she ... Ju ... ((takes the paper and writes the name of

[8] sister)) home afterwards.

[9] Ig: Your sister Julia helped you after the accident! And who do you live with today?

[10] Ma: He... ((picks up the paper and writes his nephew's name)) does oh... ((gesture

[11] indicating that he wears a tie))

[12] Ig: Daniel, it's your nephew! Is he studying? What's he doing? Law?

[13] Ma: yeah ... her too, at the front.

[14] Ig: Daniel's mother? Do they live across the street?

[15] Ma: no ... (Zubreski ... Ol ... Ga

[16] ((write name on paper))

[17] Ig: So, now I understand, Olga is Daniel's mother, and she doesn't live here. His other [18] sister lives with him, in the house opposite.

(...)

Data 2 / writing

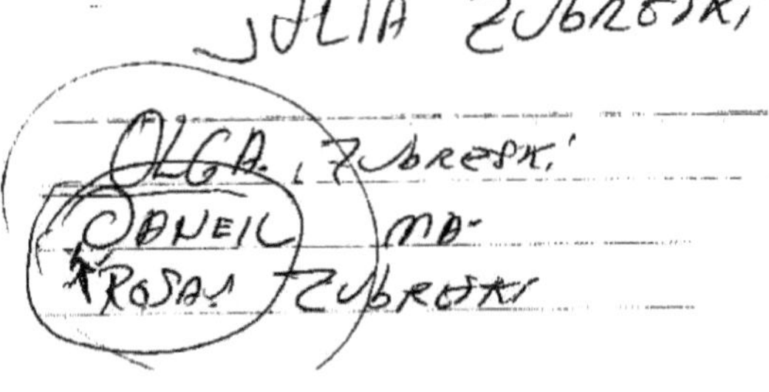

This episode demonstrates the interactive situation that results from the use of photographs, as well as the discursive conception present in working with Ma to restructure her language. It is clear to see how the dialogic situation allows the subject to act on the language, and how it is (re)elaborated. Ma assumes herself as a historical and social subject when she tells her story. Ma's difficulty with names is evident in this episode, for example in *[2] - "I had a business".* In this episode, it is clear that Ma's linguistic system is being (re)elaborated.

It's interesting to note that in order to describe the names of all his family members, he first uses the surname "*Zubreski*" and then writes down the names of his family members. In the case of "*Rosa*'s" name, he first writes it in the movable alphabet with the help of Ig and then puts it down on paper.

This episode and the writings produced by Ma reveal his participation in the interlocutive situation, the constitution of meaning is given by orality and writing and, in these dialogic situations, we see the different ways in which the aphasic places himself as a subject in language, in communication, in interaction. Here, writing ends up being another way of saying things.

3.ºEpisode (07/05/08)

Still using photographs and personal accounts, this discursive genre was used in several sessions because it was a genre that aroused greater interest in the subject and facilitated interaction between Ig and Ma. In this episode, Ma talks about his daughters and the process of separating from his ex-wife.

Data 3/orality

[1] Ig: You have two daughters, right?

(Ma picks up the paper and starts writing her daughters' names)

[2] Ma: Mari ... no ... Kessia and Ju... Julia ... Juliane

[3] Ig: Mari is his ex-wife

(takes the paper on which he has written his ex-wife's name and crosses it out)

[4] Ma: I gave ... Everything

(gestures money and writes the amount on the paper)

[5] Ig: Is that the part you'll have to pay her for? That's what's making you nervous, that the pressure is rising.

[6] Ma: oh ... all that!

(write down your pressure)

Data 3 / writing

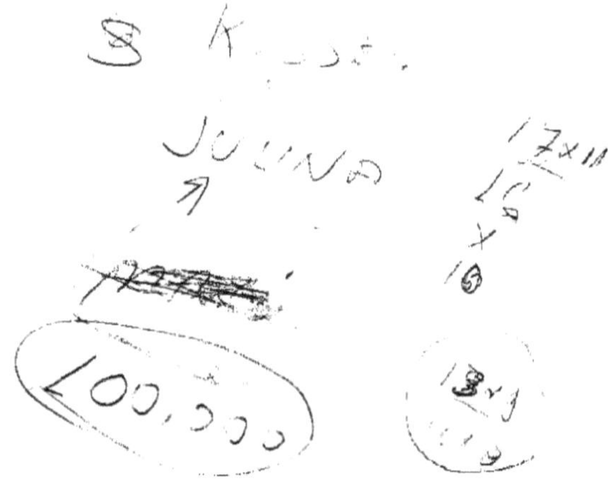

It's interesting to note that on that day Ma was very angry with his ex-wife because of the separation proceedings, so much so that he wrote "*Mari*" (his wife's name) and crossed it out. He then describes the amount she is asking for the division of assets (100,000).

The writing here shows Ma's irritation. As he writes, he puts more force into the pen, crosses out and circles the values and names, showing the same irritation as his speech. And next to these writings the numbers 17 x 11 and 16 x 10 are the values of his pressure when he was talking to the lawyer and his wife.

The construction of mutual knowledge helped Ig to establish previously shared assumptions

(Ig already knew his daughters' names and the story of the separation) through verbal interaction. This allowed Ma to make use of linguistic resources in discursive practice. Coudry explains that: "The intersubjective relationship (seeking to know each other reciprocally, we are attentive to all the signs, even non-verbal, with which we can initially relate, integrating all the participants in the process, elaborating together "conversational rules") creates the conditions of interaction, not as a limit of discursive events but as the place where they can occur." (COUDRY, 1986, p.82)

The interactive situations combined with the intersubjective relationship referred to by Coudry may not provide a syntactic fluency in Ma's discourse, but they certainly contribute to a discursive fluency that involves "aspects of interaction and textuality far beyond the syntactic phenomenon" (MARCUSCHI, 2001c, p.61).

4.° Episode (28/05/08)

In the hope of becoming an interlocutor, subject Ma resumes habits that were present in his life before the neurological event, such as renewing his driver's license, using the internet, traveling, among others.

Ma's interest in renewing her driver's license was a relevant factor in creating strategies for both assessment and therapeutic intervention. With the aim of creating dialogic discursive situations, as well as broadening the interaction between the interlocutors, at the beginning of the activities we worked on traffic signs, car manuals, maps, among others.

The episode that will be described is a conversation between Ig and Ma, about Ma's concern about renewing her driver's license.

Data 4 / orality

[1] Ma: It's hard for me to say

[2] Ig: Say what you want?What paper to write on? It's a book

[3] Ma: Yes, it's bad to talk

[4] Ig: What do you want to do?

[5] Ma: I'd go and see, I don't know!

[6] Ig: Take off Ca ... Ca..

[7] Ma: ((picks up old driver's license)) I used to say, I don't know how to speak, I know everything else

[8] but I can't speak. I know everything here, but I don't know how to talk

[9] Ig: This book here, it's a transit book and we're going to start working here on the

[10] therapies.

Dice 4 / drawing

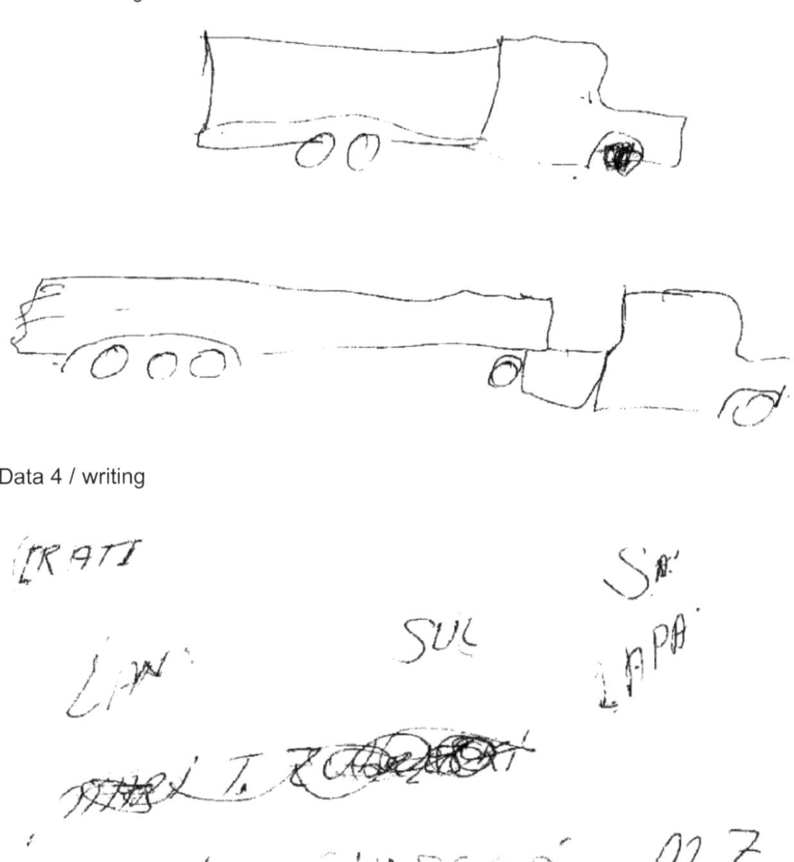

Data 4 / writing

In this session, Ig brings various resources to therapy, such as maps, a movable alphabet and pictures of traffic signs. At the beginning of the therapy, Ma tells us about the need to renew his driving license (orality data) and with the therapist's questions during the interaction, he tells us, with the help of the map, the cities he has traveled to (Irati, Laranjeiras do Sul, Sao Paulo, Lapa, Chapecó). These words are written down because they are the cities that Ma had difficulty saying the name of when looking at the map of Brazil.

The city Laranjeiras do Sul, he only writes "*Lan*" and manages to say the rest of the word, so he gives up writing the word altogether, because the importance at this point is not the writing of the word but the fluency of his oral speech (important for both him and Ig).

In Figure 4, the drawing of the trucks, Ma relates her journeys to the different types of vehicles she has driven. When he started traveling before his marriage, he only drove small trucks and made short journeys. Over time and with his knowledge of the road, he traveled to far-flung places, such as the whole of southern Brazil or from São Paulo to Amapà, which began to lead to arguments with his wife, which he explains when he writes her name and, during his oral speech, crosses it out, which even led to their separation.

The use of writing in this episode also included drawing. It's worth pointing out that Ma was showing the need to use the written modality of language, as well as drawing, to interact with her interlocutor Ig, when she had difficulties with orality. Ma used writing as an interlocutive resource in different discursive situations. These writings have no meaning if analyzed individually, i.e. the part of the oral interaction in which they were produced. They would be a pile of papers on which only fragments of Ma's writing could be seen, without constituting a semantic unit.

Ma's writing loses its fragmented character when it is revealed in the context of orality. In other words, Ma's writing reflects meaning when it is placed in a socio-communicative context. You can see in the situation described how this occurs [2] when Ig asks Ma if he wants to use writing to describe what he would like to improve with therapy. He agrees and draws a picture of a truck, which represents the usefulness of his driving license, and in an informal way uses writing and speech at the same time to answer the question he has been asked. Both written and spoken language are used by Ma in his response attempts, which indicates an interdependence between them in this production condition.

5th Episode (04/06/08)

In this episode, Ma's transit through the two modalities of language is clear. With visual support and contextualized words, texts from DETRAN's traffic law book were read orally.

Data 5 / orality

[1] Ig: First let's read this text about the car, you're used to it.Let [2] me find it here.

[3] Ma: Here ... is ... bad to say ... It's bad to speak. It's not allowed here,

[4] You can't pass here. I know everything, but I can't speak. I know everything

[5] Ig: So let's do it this way, I'll read it with you, OK?

[6] Ma: This one...

[7] Ig: What is it?

[8] Ma: I can't speak... I know

[9] Ig: What does the car need? Look at this one?

[10] Ma: mo ..

[11] Ig: Tor and energy ...

((picks up paper and writes motor))

[12] Ig: Exactly

[13] Ma: So, I know, I see, I know everything ... but it's hard to talk about.

[14] Ig: I see, you're telling me that when you see it, it's easier, to say that it's [15] difficult, so let's try to do it like this ... let's talk about what's going on

[16] written.

((picks up the text and looks at it))

[17] Ma: car ... this ... like this oh ((write the make and model of your car))

[18] Ig: Your car is a Gol, mine is too! And let's put together what it needs [19] to run, as it says in the text.

((Ig and Ma use the movable alphabet to assemble the words and then he copies them))

Data 5 / writing

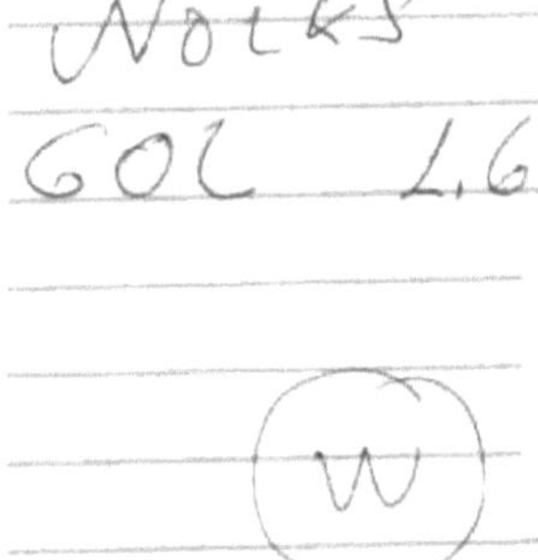

The car:

The automobile is nothing more than an assembly made up of several systems in which an engine transforms and turns mechanical energy in order to move it.

The engine can be either internal combustion or electric, and the former, which is more common, will be the object of our study. The internal combustion engine needs ignition, power, cooling, exhaust and lubrication systems to work.

The vehicle's speed and direction of travel are controlled by the gearbox and engine speed.

Knowledge and understanding of how a machine works makes it easier to use, maintain and prevent poor performance.

This makes it easier to detect possible faults, carry out efficient maintenance and make proper use of a vehicle when you understand how it works.

Source: http://www.detran.pr.gov.br

ÓLEO DE FREIO, DO MOTOR

HIDRÁULICO:

ÁGUA DO RADIADOR

As in the previous session, reported in episode 4, the strategy of maps and the discussion about trucks and journeys produced a broadening of Ma's discourse, and the interaction was effective. In the next session, Ig tried to follow up the theme of "journeys" and "cars" and brought traffic signs and the driver's handbook issued by DETRAN to therapy.

We began our work with Ma telling us that he wanted to

change his car, then Ig suggests that they read the text about the car and discuss it.

In the course of the discussion, Ma tells us about the make of his car. In his oral speech, he has difficulty naming it, so he resorts to writing (data 5/writing). This passage is important because it shows how the subject manages to use writing to support his oral speech, and even though he still has difficulty with the lexical access of words, he manages to interact with Ig and relate the events.

Reading the text "The automobile", the part where it says: "(...) *when you understand how a motor vehicle works, it becomes easier to detect possible malfunctions* (...)"; Ig asks Ma what it takes for a car to work well, Ma tells him and uses the drawings that are just below in the traffic book.

When he tries to explain the items to Ig, the difficulties of lexical access appear, so Ig guides him to assemble the words in the movable alphabet and then write them down on paper (the writing reported in data 5).

In the episode highlighted above, we can clearly see the impact of the difficulty of lexical access on contiguity. The therapist uses resources such as paper, pen and the movable alphabet to help him understand the text. When he can't access the lexicon, he uses the writing of the word as an expressive resource. It is worth noting in this episode the effort that subject Ma makes to try to fix names in any way, such as using the movable alphabet and rewriting the words and then trying to read them.

Another important point is the therapist's use of a different textual genre. In the personal account genre, Ma's speech was less difficult to access lexically.

Analyzing Ma's episodes 4 and 5 and considering the issues of the speech-writing relationship and, consequently, the textual genres worked on (personal account and informative text) and the manipulation carried out by the aphasic, it was possible to see that genres that are a little more formal, in the case of the informative text, require more elaboration in the discourse, in the case of Ma, and consequently more difficulties related to his aphasia, which occurs with the text about the car, as it is a slightly more elaborate genre and requires a more complex abstraction.

However, the personal account, which was more communicative in nature and which Ma dealt with on a daily basis, is more spontaneous and informal, and was more easily used by Ma, allowing her to communicate and say what she was thinking or feeling.

The contextualization of discursive genres is another important factor. For Ma, writing to communicate is part of his daily life and an essential task that really makes sense to him.

6th episode (13/08/08)

This therapy session takes place after he returns from his vacation at the clinic, trying to maintain interaction with Ma, Ig brings phrases from the truck to the discussion.

Data 6 / orality

[1] Ig: Shall we try to read this sentence? Try to understand it

[2] Ma: ((*looks at the sentence and reads silently))* E..E..I ... se... E..I look ... I know [3] .. ma.. ma ... L3 num... I look here and think ((*gets emotional*))

[4] Ig : Then let's go!

[5] Ma: Po.. Because it's bad to say. Me...Me ... num...

((*hand gestures of going forward))*

[6] Ig: Let's see here ... VI...

[7] Ma: Vi...DA

[8] Ig : Now let's try another one! A..Pe..NAS

[9] Ma: ((*repeats along))* NAS

[10] Ig: APE... APE ... NAS

[11] Ma: ONLY ... Just one of ... What's it like?

[12] Ig : DA ...

[13] Ma: What's it like?

[14] Ig : Look at me DA ... DA ... Oh! D and A .. DA ... now the first letter of your [15] name? What is it?

[16] Ma: Mario!

[17] Ig: So oh! Just a DA...?

[18] Ma: Lady! Mâ ... mâ ... and this one? What's this one's name?

[19] Ig : N and O ... oh ... NO ((*Ma looks at the therapist and keeps quiet)*) NO... so

[20] Shall we? No..

[21] Ma: BA ... RA ... LHO

[22] Ig : BARALHO

[23] Ma: Dâo ... no ...

[24] Ig : Vi... iii

[25] Ma: LIFE .... EN... CON... TREI

[27] Ma: The woman ...

[28] Ig : Only

[29] Ma: ((Repeats along)) Just one of the ... range...

[30] Ig : From...

[31] Ma: Lady ... Yeah ... this one, or like this ((*Makes the Q and K symbol, from the letters of the*

[32] *deck))*

[33] Ig : That's what it's like...

[34] Ma: Yeah, I said ... like oh!?

(...)

Data 6 / writing

'In the BARALHO OF LIFEJ I FOUND ARENAS AÌDAMA! "

During the session, first there was silent reading because of Ma's difficulty in understanding some words when they were unfamiliar to him. Then Ma and Ig began reading together, with the therapist reading a few words and Ma completing and continuing the sentence. After this, a second reading took place. During the recording, Ma became more independent after the second reading.

As he himself says in other passages, when the word becomes familiar, reading aloud is more fluent. After the reading, what was implicit in the sentences was discussed and the meaning was reached together with the therapist. Inserted in interactive and dialogic situations, in which the social rules of the language game originate in the practice of language, Ma is gradually reconstructing his language and constituting himself once again as an active subject in the interlocutions.

For another two months Ig brought truck-related topics to the session, strategies such as: more truck phrases, trucker jokes, maps, road guides. During this time, we can clearly see what Fàvero (2002) says: "a spoken text is directly linked to the way the interactional activity is organized between the participants" (p.22). And in Ma's case, the writing also follows this line, it is organized according to the situation of interaction and, as in orality, this organization has as its final product interpretative decisions, inferred from cognitive and cultural preconstructions, accessed at the moment of the conversational activity.

Ig is the investigator and plays the role of mediator, producing or favoring dialogic situations, playing the role of facilitator of discursive exchanges throughout the session, creating "amplifying" responses. After reading it together, as shown in Figure 7, Ig and Ma discuss the meaning of the sentence and Ma recounts some events related to her travels with some of the women she met.

The speech therapist should introduce the aphasic patient to different discursive genres, as this circulation makes it possible to finish the statements better, giving the patient greater autonomy.

7° episode (26/11/08)

On this day, as it would be the last session of the year, Ig had prepared another strategy related to Christmas and the end of the year celebrations, but Ma arrived at the session carrying the "Gazeta do povo" (local newspaper) and saying that she would like to read the report.

Data 7 / orality

[1] Ma: What's this? ((*points to the word*))

[2] Ig: Young man!

[3] Ma: Young man. And this? I know everything... this one, this one... I didn't [4] know anything about L4! I look, but it's hard to say!

[5] Ig: Now from this article that we've already read and these words that you already know, [6] you're going to L6 try to write here! Just the ones you crossed out.

[7] Ma: It could be...

[8] Ig: Let's try reading! Do you want to read it?

[9] Ma: Speak first!

[10] Ig: Number ...

[11] Ma: What's it like?

[12] Ig: Number ...

[13] Ma: The number ...

[14] Ig: Crescent

[15] Ma: Crescent of ... Bo ... bordage ...

[16] Ig: Errors

[17] Ma: Errors in bo ....

[18] Ig: Approaches ...

[19] Ma: Police approach

[20] Ig: Police

[21] Ma: This one?

[22] Ig: The ... affects ... ((*tries to repeat and can't)*) Affects ...

[23] Ma: AFETA faze... family

[24] Ig: And it generates i..

[25] Ma: Insecurity in the dust ... dust ...

[26] Ig: Population

[27] Ma: Population ban ... BA.. BA...

[28] Ig: Brazilian

[29] Ma: Brazilian

[30] Ig: expert ... man ...

[31] Ma: characterizing the a... What's it like?

[32] Ig: increase in ....

[33] Ma: approaches

[34] Ig: e.e .....

[35] Ma: wrong

[36] Ig: and suggests ...

[37] Ma: need ((silence))

[38] Ig: tra . ((asks to look at your mouth))

[39] Ma: psychological treatment ...

[40] Ig: psychological

[41] Ma: That's a difficult word...

[42] Ig: ((laughs))

[43] Ma: for the military

[44] Ig: military police

[45] Ma: How do you speak?

[46] Ig: in ... ves ... researcher

[47] Ma: instead

[48] Ig: Oh! ((speaks slowly)) researchers

[49] Ma: investigators ... military police

[50] Ig: civil investigators.

(...)

Data 7 / writing

The growing number of errors in police approaches affects families and creates insecurity among the Brazilian population. The increase in mistaken police approaches suggests the need for psychological treatment for military police officers, says the civil police investigator, who defends the training.

Source: Gazeta do Povo newspaper

POLICIAIS FAMILIAS INSEGURANÇA BRASILEIRA

First Ig read the headline and Ma showed interest. Then he was asked to read and mark the words he knew.

This first reading allowed Ma to familiarize himself with the text and the words, making it easier to read aloud. This dynamic was used because in several sessions he reported that when he read silently first, comprehension was made easier.

We then discussed the article and read it aloud together. At the beginning of the reading, Ma also asked the therapist for help, as shown in [9].

In [3] and [4] Ma told the therapist that there were several words in the text that he knew and that he couldn't read after the accident.

Even though they were still reading together in this strategy, Ma showed more autonomy in reading, completing the next words of what was being read.

The writing shown in data 7 are the words that Ma read in the report and identified as "*known words*". I then asked him to copy them and then read them separately to gain a better understanding of the journalistic text.

It is possible to see the improvement in Ma's language, as she uses orality and writing more and more efficiently in joint productions. Ma gradually overcomes his linguistic difficulties, from the perspective of constitutive language, establishing himself as a subject. The linguistic-discursive approach allows the aphasic to play their part in the turns of interlocution. In this respect, Coudry states: "*I assume, as I have reiterated, that the dialogical process characterizes language and is the place of constitution for other modes of verbal action.*" (COUDRY, 1986, p.76).

8th episode (09/04/09)

The interrelationship established by Ma between orality and writing proves the initial hypothesis of the role of the informal use of writing in the therapeutic process with aphasic subjects. This can be seen in the following episode, in which Ig begins the session by asking how Ma's weekend had been, which she says had been very good; she then begins to tell him about a conversation she had with a friend, with whom she hadn't spoken since before the stroke, on the telephone. It's worth noting that Ma manages to keep the conversation flowing without having to resort to drawing or written language.

Data 8/orality

[1] Ig: You were at home.

[2] Ma:Everything's fallen down, right? And a man who's been my neighbor for many years... how's everything going?

[3] Ig: Did you call him?

[4] Ma: So, I... all right... I had something of theirs, of hers, right? Which I have very well, I was able to say everything.

[5] Ig: With him on the phone?

[6] Ma: Yes. But what about... when I know and I can't do it anymore.

[7] Ig: Ah, then he asked you, what did you have?

[8] Ma: Yes, everything, more .....

[9] Ig: You explained everything, then when he asked, you couldn't speak anymore.

[10] Ma: But there's nothing...

[11] Ig: Then you didn't get anything else. And because then you stopped, you left the speech.

[12] Ma: Exactly.

[13] Ig: And you had to think in order to answer and then that blocked your speech.

[14] Ma: Yes.

[15] Ig: Why was it that while you were talking to him you were able to say everything?

[16] Ma: Everything, almost everything, right? I was talking.

[17] Ig: Did you tell him what you had? Everything?

[18] Ma: No, he said I had.

[19] Ig: Oh, he knew.

[20] Ma: Yes.

[21] Ig: He had heard about it.

Data 8 / writing

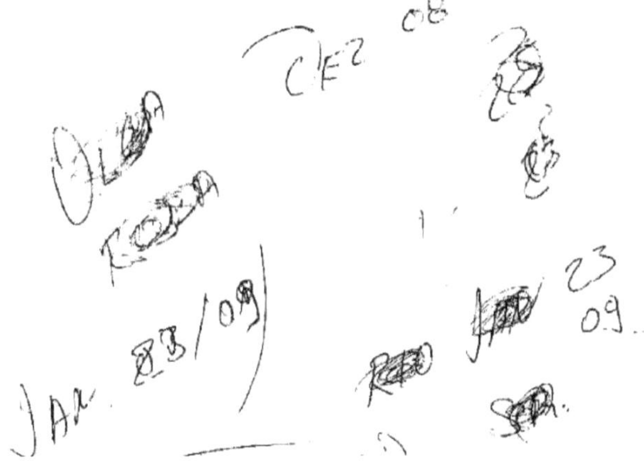

This account described in data 8 is interesting, as it shows Ma's account of a conversation he had with a friend on the phone. While he was describing it to Ig, he picked up the pen and paper and began to write and rework his writing on his own.

In line 2, when he wants to explain that an old friend called him "*He's a man who's been a neighbor of mine for many years*", he writes down *the names* of his sisters, because they also knew this *man. he writes the* names of his sisters, because they also knew this man. By putting their names on the paper, he has more confidence in telling Ig what happened.

This friend currently lives in Rio de Janeiro and still keeps in touch with Ma's sisters, but after the accident, they spoke to each other on the phone.

This was of great importance to Ma, as it showed him that he can interact with other people, even outside the therapy session and without the therapist's help.

Ma's evolutionary process and his steps towards reconstituting his language appear very clearly to him. The way in which he reworks his speech in the different discursive dialogic situations to which Ma has been subjected shows him at this point how he has managed to restructure himself linguistically, constituting himself as a historical and social subject.

Ma regained the security to maintain an interactive dialogic situation, much more marked in the interaction with Ig; managing in a way to face his linguistic difficulties, trying to occupy his place in the dialog, in order to face his biggest barrier, anomie.

Given that Ma's image of himself as a speaker/writer directly affected his discursive production, we tried to intervene in this relationship during the therapies. At times, Ma stopped comparing his speech before with now, repeating several times that "*before he knew and now he doesn't*". This negative relationship between Ma and language can be mitigated by the use of writing. This seems to have helped him establish a better interaction with others, giving him the means to act in writing when he lacked words in oral interaction.

It is understood from this case that when the social practices of reading and writing are taken into account in the speech therapy clinical process, the aphasic subject expands their possibilities of using symbolic resources to position themselves as the author of their own discourse.

5 FINAL CONSIDERATIONS

The purpose of seeking answers to the concerns that arose during the researcher's undergraduate years proved to be opportune, especially since it was these questions that guided the research and made it possible to fulfill the proposed objective.

With regard to the first concern raised about the functioning of the language of aphasic subjects, it was possible to see from discursive neurolinguistics that far beyond understanding just how language works, it is necessary to understand what resources each aphasic uses to interact with others through language. In order to understand these resources, a series of historical and social factors are taken into account, not only for the aphasic but also for the non-aphasic who is part of the interaction process.

Always bearing in mind that this interaction doesn't have a predetermined meaning, but it's the moment that surrounds it that determines that meaning.

The second concern is related to the limitations and linguistic-discursive specificities of aphasics. It is possible to state, based on the perspective taken during the course of the research, that the focus during the written language therapy process with the aphasic subject changes. In other words, don't look at what the subject can't achieve and their difficulties, but rather at what they are producing, their potential and the intersubjective resources they use to achieve interaction with others.

Having understood the issues described above, the elaboration of written language therapy must take into account the social practices of reading and writing of the aphasic subject and the intersubjective characteristics of each subject.

It is up to the speech therapist to approach different discursive genres that are related to the subject's daily life, topics of interest that promote an interactive process, in which it is possible to highlight the aphasic's potential and show them the resources they can use to overcome the difficulties resulting from the brain injury.

It is also the therapist's role to discover resources, such as a mobile alphabet, photos, maps, among others, which help and benefit the moment of interaction between the therapist and the subject. In other words, the speech therapist must play the role of mediator and participant in the interaction, highlighting the potential that the aphasic subject is realizing.

This whole process of mediation and interaction is described in the longitudinal follow-up of Ma's case, shown in the sequence of episodes presented in this research. The analysis of Ma's data in these episodes allows us to observe significant progress in her language, highlighting the importance of the theoretical-methodological position maintained by Ig, who played a dual role in this study: that of researcher and Ma's interlocutor. The situations of interaction experienced between the interlocutors led Ma to assume a more active position in the dialog. In the course of the episodes, it becomes clear how Ma starts to operate more and more on her difficulties, increasing the extent of her oral productions, reducing comparisons with her speech before and after the traumatic brain injury.

The use of visual resources during this therapeutic process had great results in Ma's case, due to the particularities of this subject with the functioning of his language, and shows that it is up to the therapist to identify the necessary resources that each subject uses to (re)organize his language, bearing in mind that each subject is unique.

In these interactive situations, Ma acquired the conditions to expand his possibilities of operating with language. She began to question, to make inferences, to organize accounts of her own life, so as to occupy her place in the discourse in a more meaningful way, assuming herself as a subject.

Ma's use of writing appears to be linked to her social need - to renew her driver's license - and also as an expressive resource inserted in dialogical interactive situations.

Finally, it should be emphasized that enunciative-discursive neurolinguistics and the concept of literacy are essential for guiding therapeutic work with aphasic subjects. The aphasic subject's interest in the activity of meaning and re-signifying language is evident. During the therapeutic process, they use all the resources at their disposal (speaking, writing, gestures, drawings) to interact with a therapist who is attentive and willing to insert themselves into the discursive chain established between them. Therefore, intersubjective activities and interaction with others, especially an attentive and sensitive therapist, are effective means of overcoming linguistic-discursive difficulties and re-signifying the language of aphasic subjects.

REFERENCES

ANDRADE, V. M. Neuropsicologia Hoje, Sâo Paulo, Artes Médicas. 2004.

ANTUNHA, E. L. G. Neuropsychological assessment in childhood. In: V. B. Oliveira and N. A. Bossa (org.), Avaliaçâo psicopedagógica da criança de 0 a 6 anos. Rio de Janeiro: vozes, 2002.

ANTONIO, B. S. M. *Interdependent relationships between orality and writing in a case of aphasia.* Master's thesis - Federal University of Paranà. Curitiba, 2004.

ARANTES, L. Diagnòstico e clinica de linguagem. - Sâo Paulo: s.n., Tese (Doutorado) Pontificia Universidade Católica de Sâo Paulo. 2005.

ARDILA, A. *Aphasias.* Department of Communication Sciences and Disorders, Florida International University, Miami, Florida, USA. 2006.

BAKHTIN, M. *The genres of discourse.* IN: BAKHTIN, M. *Estética a criaçao verbal.* Sâo Paulo: Martins Fontes. 1997.

BASSEY, M. On the nature of research in education. Research Intelligence, n.36, p 1618, 1990.

BAGNO, M. *Preconceito linguistico:* o que é, como se faz. 27 ed. Sâo Paulo: Loyola, 2003.

CARTHERY-GOULART, M. T., & PARENTE, M. A. M. P. Reading and writing and ageing. In M. A. M. P. Parente (Ed.), *Cognition and ageing* (pp. 191202). Porto Alegre, RS: Artmed. 2006.

CORRÊA, M.L.G. *O modo heterogêneo de constituiçao da escrita.* Sâo Paulo: Martins Fontes, 2004.

COUDRY, M. I. H. *Diàrio de Narciso : discourse and aphasia.* Sâo Paulo: Martins Fontes, 1986/ 1988.

ELLIS, A. W. YOUNG, A. W. Human Cognitive Neuropsychology. London: Lawrence Erlbaum Associates. 1988.

FLOSI, L.C.L.; The Relationship between the Dynamics of Oral Language and Writing and Gestures in Aphasia. Campinas/ IEL - 04/2003

FONSECA, S. C. *O afàsico na clinica da linguagem.* (Doctoral thesis). Sâo Paulo: s.n. Pontifical Catholic University of São Paulo. 2002.

FRANCHI, C. Linguagem atividade constitutiva. **Cadernos de Estudos Lingüisticos**, Sâo Paulo, v.22, p.9-39, 1977-1992.

FREUD, S. **Mal estar na civilizaçao**. Rio de Janeiro, Imago, Standard Editions, Volume XXI, 1969

FREIRE, F. M. O. *A agenda màgica.* Thesis (Doctorate in Linguistics) Institute of Language Studies, State University of Campinas, Campinas, 2005.

GARCEZ, L. H. do C. *A escrita e o Outro: os modos de participaçao na construção do texto.* Brasilia:

Editora Universidade de Brasilia, 1998.

GIL, R. *Neuropsycholoogie*. 3ª Ed. Parins: Masson. 2003.

GOLDSTEIN, K. Language and language disturbances. New York: Grune & Stratton. 1948.

HÉCAEN, H., & ALBERT, M.L. Human neuropsychology. New York: Wiley. 1978.

INFANTE, U. Texto: Leitura e escritas. São Paulo: Scipione, 2000.

JAKUBOVICZ, R. & MEINBERG, R. *Introduction to Aphasia: Elements for Diagnosis and Therapy.* Rio de Janeiro: Revinter, 1985

KRISTENSEN, C. H.; ALMEIDA, R. M. M.; GOMES, W. B. *Historical development and methodological foundations of cognitive neuropsychology.* IN: Revista Psicologia: Reflexâo e critica. Vol. 14 n° 2. Porto Alegre, 2001

LURIA, A. R. *Fundamentals of Neuropsychology. Sao Paulo. Editora da USP. 1984.*

MACEDO, H. O. O *processo de refacçao textual escrita na linguagem escrita de sujeitos afàsicos.* Thesis (doctorate in linguistics) - Institute of Language Studies, State University of Campinas, Campinas (SP): [s.n.], 2006.

MAINGUENEAU, D. **Novas tendências em anàlise do discurso.** Campinas: Pontes/Unicamp, 1989

MARCUSCHI, L. A. *Letramento e oralidade no contexto das prâticas sociais e eventos comunicativos.* IN: SIGNORINI, I. (org.) *Investigando a relação oral/escrito.* Campinas (SP): Mercado de Letras, 2001

MAYRINK-SABINSON, M. L.; FIAD, R.; ABAURRE, µ. B., **Scenes in the acquisition of writing. The subject and working with the text**. Campinas (SP), 2002.

MEY, J. *As vozes da sociedade: seminàrios de pragmàtica*. Campinas (SP): Mercado de Letras, 2001.

MOREIRA, H. and CALEFFE M. B. Pesquisa educacional: reflexôes sobre os paradigmas de pesquisa. In: FINGER, A. P. et al. Educaçâo: caminhos e perspectivas. Curitiba: Champagnt, 2006).

MURDOCH, B. E. Boston and Lûria Aphasia Syndromes. Rio de Janeiro, 1997.

NOPPEY, U. and WALLESCH, C. W. *Language and cognition* - Kurt Goldstein's. Theory of semantics. Brain and Cognition, v. 44, p. 367 - 386, 2000.

NOVAES-PINTO, R. C. and SANTANA, A. P. Semiology of aphasia: a critical discussion. In. MANCOPES, R. and SANTANA, A. P. (org). Perspectives on the aphasia clinic: The subject and discourse. Revinter, 2009.

PARENTE, M. A. M. P. Conduta Clinica. In A. R. Lecours & M. A. M. P. Parente (eds), Dyslexia:

implicações do sistema de escrita do português (PP. 85 - 105). Porto Alegre: Artes Médicas, 1997).

PINHEIRO, A. M. V. Reading and spelling development in Brazilian Portuguese Reading & Writing 7 (1), 111 - 138, 1995.

ORTIZ, K. Z. *Acquired Neurological Disorders*. 1 ed. Sâo Paulo: Editora Manole, 2005.

ORTIZ, K. Z.; ARAUJO, A. A.; PRIETO, F. F. *Clinical cases of acquired reading and writing disorders: dyslexia and agraphia.* IN: ORTIZ, K. Z. (org) *Acquired Neurological Disorders*. 1ª. Sâo Paulo: Editora Manole, 2005.

ROJO, R. *Didactic modeling and planning:* two forgotten teacher practices? IN: KLEIMAN, A. A *formação do professor: perspectivas da lingüistica aplicada.* Campinas (SP): Mercado das Letras, 2001.

SALLES, J.F. *The use of phonological and lexical reading routes in schoolchildren: relationships with comprehension, reading time and phonological awareness.* Master's thesis. Postgraduate Diploma in Developmental Psychology, Federal University of Rio Grande do Sul / UFRGS. Porto Alegre, RS. 2001.

SANTANA, A. P. *Escrita e afasia: a linguagem escrita na afasiologia.* São Paulo:

Plexus, 2002.

SANTANA, A. P. and MACEDO, H. O. *Aphasia, literacy practices and therapeutic implications.* IN: BERBERIAN, A. P.; MASSI, G. and ANGELIS, C. C. M. *Letramento: referência em saù e educaçao.* Sâo Paulo: Plexus, 2006.

SIGNORINI, I. Introduction. In: Investigating the oral / written relationship. Campinas (SP):

Mercado de Letras, 2001.

STREET; B. V. *Social literacies. Critical approaches to literacy in development, ethnography and education*. Harbow: Longman, 1995.

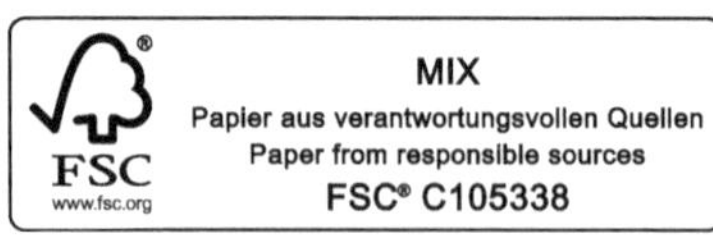

Printed by Books on Demand GmbH, Norderstedt / Germany